The Kidney-Friendly Diet

50 Easy-Prepared Recipes to Maintain Healthy Kidneys

Tiara Crocker

Table of Contents

Introduction

It is pretty important to know about the function of each organ of the body. Concerning the kidneys, their function is to eliminate the excess toxins and clean the blood. Besides, They are capable to create hormones that deal with red blood cell growth.

For all this, it is crucial to keep healthy eating habits in order to maintain the kidneys in optimal conditions and prevent different diseases related to a damaged kidney.

The present book offers 50 recipes beneficial to boost your renal capacities of helping your body to stay well with plenty of food products low in sodium and potassium.

Chapter 1: Breakfast

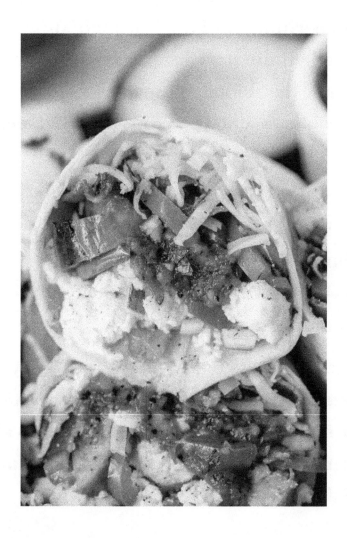

1. Breakfast Burritos with Eggs and Mexican Sausage

(Ready in about 30 minutes | Serving 3 | Difficulty: Medium)

Per serving: Kcal 320, Fat: 20 g, Net Carbs: 17 g, Protein: 16 g

Ingredients:

- 3 tortillas

- 3 beaten eggs

- 3 oz. Mexican sausage chorizo

Instructions:

1. In a skillet, fry chorizo till darkened. Then put eggs and let it cook.
2. Fill the tortillas with the mixture and roll to serve.

2. Mexican Egg and Tortilla Skillet Breakfast (Megas)

(Ready in about 20 minutes | Serving 6 | Difficulty: Easy)

Per serving: Kcal 297, Fat: 20 g, Net Carbs: 18 g, Protein: 11 g

Ingredients:

- 2 thinly sliced green onions

- 8 eggs

- 1 tsp. chili powder

- 6 oz. tortilla chips

- ¼ cup ketchup

- 2 tbsp. butter

Instructions:

1. Beat the eggs well
2. Then add ketchup, chili powder, and onion and beat again. Put it aside.

3. In a skillet, melt the butter, then sauté tortilla chips till warmed. Add the egg mixture and cook till done.

3. Easy Turkey Breakfast Burritos

(Ready in about 15 minutes | Serving 8 | Difficulty: Easy)

Per serving: Kcal 407, Fat: 24 g, Net Carbs: 21 g, Protein: 25 g

Ingredients:

- 8 shells flour burrito (6")

- ¼ cup canola oil

- 2 tbsp. chopped fresh scallions

- 8 scrambled eggs

- ¼ cup onions diced

- ¼ cup diced bell peppers

- 2 tbsp. jalapeño peppers seeded

- 2 tbsp. chopped fresh cilantro

- ½ tsp. chili powder

- ½ tsp. smoked paprika

- Meatloaf(Half Kg).

Instructions:

1. Sauté peppers, onion, meatloaf, cilantro, and scallions till translucent. Add spices and remove from heat.
2. In the other pan, add oil and eggs. Put the mixture in burritos and serve.

Chapter 2: Smoothies and Drinks

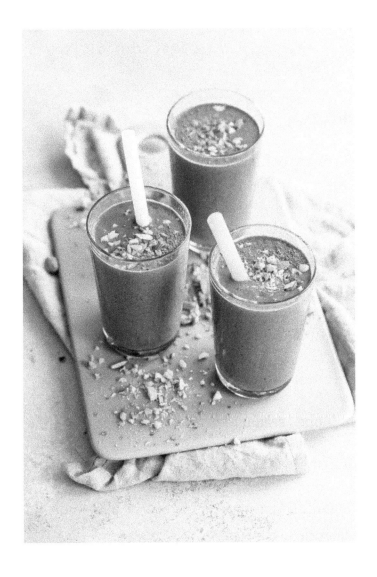

4. Chocolate Smoothie

(Ready in about 2 minutes | Serving 4 | Difficulty: Easy)

Per serving: Kcal 142, Fat: 4 g, Net Carbs: 16 g, Protein: 10 g

Ingredients:

- ¼ tsp. ground cinnamon

- 2 cups ice

- 1 pinch nutmeg

- ¼ cup milk (condensed)

- ½ cup milk (evaporated)

- 2 chocolate-flavored scoops whey protein

- Whipped cream to garnish

Instructions:

1. Blend all the ingredients except cinnamon till smooth.
2. Garnish with whipped cream and cinnamon.

5. Orange Flavored Coffee

(Ready in about 5 minutes | Serving 20 | Difficulty: Easy)

Per serving: Kcal 47, Fat: 0.8 g, Net Carbs: 9 g, Protein: 0.4 g

Ingredients:

- 1 cup Powder Coffee Mate®

- ½ tsp. orange peel dried

- ¾ cup sugar

- ½ cup instant coffee

- 1 tsp. hot water for each cup

Instructions:

1. Process all the components in the blender to make powder, then for each cup, put 2 tsp. in one cup of hot water.

6. Lemonade or Limeade Base

(Ready in about 30 minutes | Serving 10 | Difficulty: Easy)

Per serving: Kcal 108, Fat: 0 g, Net Carbs: 27 g, Protein: 0 g

Ingredients:

- 1¼ cups lime juice

- 1 ¼ cups sugar

- ½ tsp. shredded lime peel

- 2 ½ cups of water

Instructions:

1. Dissolve sugar in water over a moderate flame, then let it cool for about twenty minutes. Add the juice and peel in the sugar mix and put it in a jar, and chill. Leftover can be saved by freezing.

7. Berry Smoothie

(Ready in about 2 minutes | Serving 1 | Difficulty: Easy)

Per serving: Kcal 188, Fat: 3 g, Net Carbs: 28 g, Protein: 8 g

Ingredients:

- 2/3 cup firm silken tofu

- ¼ cup cocktail cranberry juice

- 1 tsp. vanilla extract

- ½ cup frozen raspberries, unsweetened

- ½ cup frozen blueberries, unsweetened

Instructions:

1. Blend everything till smooth. Serve and enjoy.

Chapter 3: Snacks and Sides

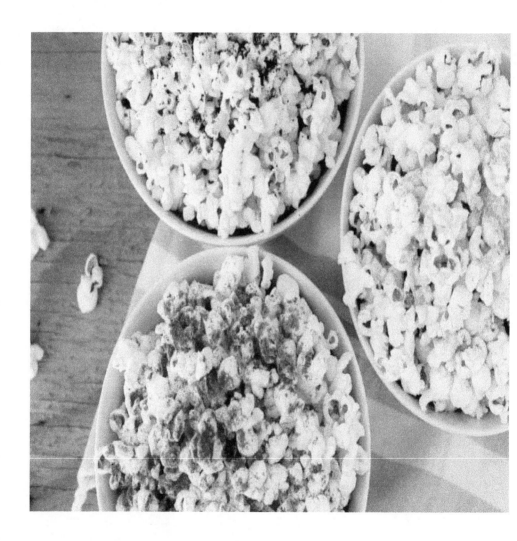

8. Popcorn 3 Ways

(Ready in about 20 minutes | Serving 3 | Difficulty: Easy)

Per serving: Kcal 275, Fat: 19 g, Net Carbs: 19 g, Protein: 3 g

Ingredients:

- 1 tsp. cinnamon

- 1 ½ tbsp. canola oil

- ¼ cup popcorn kernels

- 1 tsp. hot chili Sriracha sauce

- 1 tsp. nutritional yeast

- 4 tbsp. melted unsalted butter

- 2 tsp. granulated sugar

Instructions:

1. In a medium saucepan, pour in the canola oil and put over moderate flame.

2. Put three kernels of popcorn and place a cover on the pan that is partially broken.

3. Insert the leftover kernels, then gently shake the pan to cover the kernels in oil until all 3 kernels had popped off. Replace the pan's partially broken lid.

4. The popcorn kernels would start to pop immediately. Remove the pan from the heat as popping delays, then dump into 3 different cups.

5. Sprinkle the chili sauce in the first bowl over the popcorn and softly toss to cover.

6. Mix 2 teaspoons of melted butter with the nutritional yeast. In the second tub, brush with popcorn and throw softly to cover.

7. Combine the cinnamon and sugar with the leftover melted butter. On the 3rd bowl, sprinkle on popcorn and toss softly to cover.

8. Split each portion into 2 portions to get 1 cup of any popcorn flavor for each individual.

9. Pineapple Coleslaw

(Ready in about 10 minutes | Serving 4 | Difficulty: Easy)

Per serving: Kcal 72, Fat: 3 g, Net Carbs: 10 g, Protein: 1 g

Ingredients:

- ¼ cup Miracle Whip

- 8 oz crushed drained and unsweetened canned pineapple

- 2 cups cabbage shredded

- ¼ cup onion chopped

Instructions:

1. Combine all ingredients and refrigerate prior to serving.

10. Cauliflower in Mustard Sauce

(Ready in about 60 minutes | Serving 4 | Difficulty: Medium)

Per serving: Kcal 51, Fat: 4 g, Net Carbs: 4 g, Protein: 1 g

Ingredients:

- 2 cups flowerets cauliflower

- 1 tsp. honey

- 2 tsp. Dijon mustard

- 1 tbsp. olive oil

- 1 tbsp. + 2 tsp. white wine vinegar

- A dash black pepper

Instructions:

1. Whisk the mustard as well as the honey together; apply vinegar and after that olive oil.
2. Some seasoning to spice with. Just set aside.
3. Apply the boiling water to the cauliflower and simmer until soft.
4. Drain thoroughly.
5. With dressing, toss the cleaned, roasted cauliflower.

6. Enable 30–45 minutes to cool and serve.

11. Chicken Nuggets with Honey Mustard Sauce

(Ready in about 20 minutes | Serving 12 | Difficulty: Easy)

Per serving: Kcal 166, Fat: 8 g, Net Carbs: 17 g, Protein: 7 g

Ingredients:

- Cooking spray

- 1 tbsp. Dijon mustard

- 1 lb. chicken breast boneless pieces (32 bite-sized)

- 2 tsp. Worcestershire sauce

- ½ cup mayonnaise

- 3 cups low-sodium finely crushed cornflakes

- 1/3 cup honey

- 1 egg

- 2 tbsp. creamer liquid non-dairy

- Butter(1/2)

Instructions:

1. In a shallow cup, stir the mustard, mayo, butter, and Worcestershire sauce combined. Chill the sauce and act as a dipping sauce before the nuggets are fried.
2. Preheat the oven to 400°F.
3. Combine the non-dairy creamer and egg in an empty bowl. Crush the cornflakes and dump the crumbs into a wide bag with a ziplock.
4. Dip the chicken parts in the egg mixture, and shake to cover with cornflake crumbs in a ziplock container.
5. Bake the nuggets for fifteen min or till finished on a baking sheet coated with cooking spray.

12. BBQ Asparagus

(Ready in about 30 minutes | Serving 6 | Difficulty: Easy)

Per serving: Kcal 86, Fat: 6 g, Net Carbs: 3 g, Protein: 3 g

Ingredients:

- 2 tbsp. lemon juice

- 1-1½ tsp. black pepper

- 2-3 tbsp. EVOO

- 1-1½ lb. Asparagus

- Oil (1 cup)

Instructions:

1. In a small bowl large enough for it to fold asparagus into it, combine the black pepper, oil, and lemon juice and cover entirely with the mixture.
2. Clean the piney ends of asparagus spears and strip them. **Tip:** Keep the spear with one hand

just under the tip, and the other at the end and bend gently. Naturally, the spear can provide where woody parts finish, and the delicate asparagus begins.

3. Roll in the oil mixture and leave the asparagus in the bowl. To prevent the oil from leaking, put the tray on a platter in the fridge to marinate before the grill gets prepared.

4. Arrange the barbecue with charcoal or gas and fire over moderate flame.

5. To prevent the spears from clinging to the plate, gently spray the veggie grilling tray, any grill bucket, or piece of dense tin foil rolled into a shallow dish using olive oil mist.

6. On a veggie grilling plate, place the asparagus and spill the leftover oil from the tray onto spears.

7. Grill the asparagus until tender and start browning, regularly rotating, around 5 minutes, in the skillet or on tin foil. Move to the dish. Serve at room temp or hotter.

13. BBQ Corn on the Cob

(Ready in about 30 minutes | Serving 8 | Difficulty: Easy)

Per serving: Kcal 109, Fat: 6 g, Net Carbs: 13 g, Protein: 2 g

Ingredients:

- 1 tbsp. parmesan cheese, grated

- 3 tbsp. olive oil

- 1 tsp. dried thyme

- 4 corn cob fresh

- 1 tsp. parsley

- ½ tsp. black pepper

Instructions:

1. Husk and clean the corn (or from the product portion of the market, you can purchase 4 packaged cobs).

2. In a big enough container, combine the cheese, oil, parsley, thyme, and black pepper to fold corn into it and cover it entirely with the mixture.

3. Drop the maize in the combination and roll to cover the corn completely.

4. Put all the maize on a dense aluminum foil sheet in the middle.

5. To build a tray, fold up the sides of the foil surface to make sure that no room is left for oil to spill onto the grill.

6. Over medium flame, put a foil sheet on grill, then grill for 20 mins, rotating when browning is finished on either side.

Chapter 4: Soups

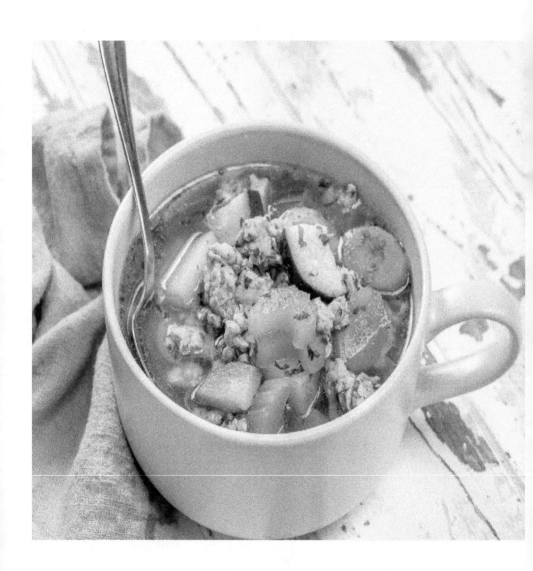

14. Mediterranean Soup Jar

(Ready in about 15 minutes | Serving 1 | Difficulty: Easy)

Per serving: Kcal 222, Fat: 10 g, Net Carbs: 20 g, Protein: 7 g

Ingredients:

- ½ cup coleslaw mix

- 1 tbsp. ricotta cheese whole milk

- 1/3 cup canned chickpeas without salt

- ½ tbsp. herb blend seasoning

- ½ cup onion strips and bell pepper

- ½ tsp. black pepper

- 1/8 tsp. pepper flakes

- 1 tsp. EVOO

- 3 large black olives reduced-sodium

- 5 oz. hot water

Instructions:

1. Cut the olives into pieces. Get the chickpeas rinsed.

2. Place all components in the 16-oz. glass jar in the order mentioned.

3. To cook and eat, refrigerate till available.

4. Detach the container from the fridge after 15 minutes until you are about to feed.

5. To mix, add 5 ounces of hot water into the container, shut the lid, and shake. Let the ingredients set for 2 minutes in an unopened pot.

6. Put the contents of the jar into a large deep container. Enjoy!

15. Cream of Chicken Wild Rice Asparagus Soup

(Ready in about 40 minutes | Serving 8 | Difficulty: Medium)

Per serving: Kcal 295, Fat: 11 g, Net Carbs: 25 g, Protein: 21 g

Ingredients:

- ½ cup onion

- 1 cup carrots

- 3 garlic cloves

- ½ tsp. pepper

- ¼ cup butter unsalted

- 2 cups asparagus

- ½ tsp. salt

- ¼ tsp. nutmeg

- 4 cups unenriched and unsweetened almond milk

- Bay leaf

- ½ cup flour

- 4 cups chicken broth low-sodium

- ½ cup vermouth extra dry

- ½ tsp. thyme

- ¾ cup wild rice and long grain blend

- 2 cups chicken cooked

Instructions:

1. As per pack instructions, prepare long grain as well as wild rice mix, eliminating salt as well as spices container, if included.
2. Take away the skillet from the heat and let the rice sit, encased, for another 15 minutes. Put aside and quit to calm off.
3. Cut the carrots, asparagus, and onion into cubes. Garlic to mince.

4. Melt butter in the Dutch oven and cook the onion and garlic till soft. Add carrots, spices, and herbs. Keep cooking until tender, over moderate flame.
5. Mix in flour and cook for 10 minutes over low heat, stir occasionally.
6. Toss in 4 cups of vermouth and chicken broth. Stir to combine, using a cord whisk.
7. Dice into tiny chunks the chicken. Add the chicken and asparagus and start adding almond milk to the soup. For 20 minutes, simmer.
8. Fold in the rice prepared, and serve.

16. Maryland's Eastern Shore Cream of Crab Soup

(Ready in about 30 minutes | Serving 7 | Difficulty: Easy)

Per serving: Kcal 130, Fat: 6 g, Net Carbs: 6 g, Protein: 12 g

Ingredients:

- 1 medium-sized onion

- 1/8 tsp. black pepper

- 4 cups chicken broth low-sodium

- 1 cup creamer half and half

- ½ lb. crab meat fresh lump

- 1/8 tsp. dill weed

- 2 tbsp. cornstarch

- ¼ tsp. Seasoning Old Bay®

- 1 tbsp. unsalted butter

Instructions:

1. Melt butter over medium flame in a big kettle.
2. Chop the onion, then apply it to the bath. Cook until the onion turns soft and clear, stirring.
3. Add meat from crabs. Cook for 2–3 mins, continuously stirring.
4. Bring the combination to a simmer and incorporate the chicken stock. Turn down the heat towards low.
5. In a shallow tub, mix creamer and cornstarch. Till smooth, whisk. Connect to the soup and slightly raise the flame, swirling continually until the mixture gets dense and boils.
6. For the broth, apply dill weed, seasoning, and pepper. Prepared to represent.

Chapter 5: Salads and Dressings

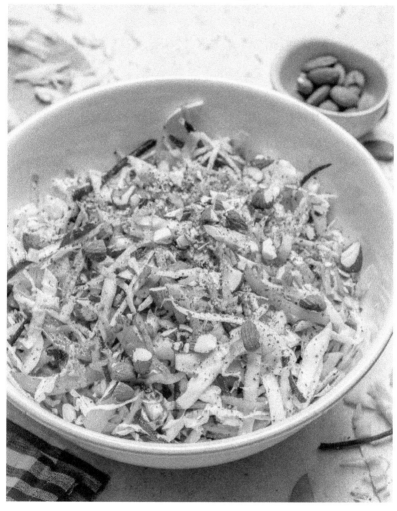

17. Chicken Fusilli Salad

(Ready in about 5 minutes | Serving 4 | Difficulty: Easy)

Per serving: Kcal 477, Fat: 29 g, Net Carbs: 31 g, Protein: 18 g

Ingredients:

Dressing:

- ¼ cup vinegar

- 1 tsp. sugar

- ½ cup olive oil

- ½ tsp. white pepper

- ¼ tsp. basil

Salad:

- 1 cup zucchini sliced

- 8 oz. diced cooked cold chicken

- ½ cup thawed peas

- 2 cups lettuce shredded

- ½ cup red pepper chopped

- 1 medium thinly sliced carrot

- 3 cups fusilli pasta, cooked

Instructions:

1. Place the seasoning ingredients in the lid jar and rattle to combine the ingredients together. Chill for 2 hours at least. Before combining with your salad, shake again.
2. In a big dish, combine the chicken, pasta, zucchini, peas, bell pepper, and carrots together.
3. Attach some dressing and tossing well. On 4 bowls, split the lettuce and cover with the salad mix.

18. Italian Eggplant Salad

(Ready in about 20 minutes | Serving 4 | Difficulty: Easy)

Per serving: Kcal 69, Fat: 5 g, Net Carbs: 6 g, Protein: 1 g

Ingredients:

- 1 small chopped onion

- 1 chopped garlic clove

- 3 cups eggplant cubed

- ½ tsp. oregano

- 3 tbsp. olive oil

- ¼ tsp. black pepper

- 1 medium chopped tomato

- 2 tbsp. wine vinegar

Instructions:

1. Cook the eggplants till they are tender and then drain. Combine black pepper, vinegar, and garlic and put all over the onion and eggplant, then put oil prior to serving.

19. Hawaiian Chicken Salad

(Ready in about 10 minutes | Serving 4 | Difficulty: Easy)

Per serving: Kcal 402, Fat: 25 g, Net Carbs: 30 g, Protein: 18 g

Ingredients:

- 2 tsp. lemon juice

- 1 ¼ cups lettuce head, shredded

- 1 cup unsweetened drained pineapple chunks

- ½ cup celery, diced

- 1 ½ cups cooked chicken, chopped

- ½ tsp. sugar

- ½ cup mayonnaise

- Paprika(1 tsp).

- A dash tabasco sauce

- ¼ tsp. pepper

Instructions:

1. Mix tabasco, mayo, lemon juice, sugar, and pepper in a separate bowl. In another bowl, add pineapple, chicken, lettuce, and celery.
2. Add the liquid mix over the chicken mix and stir. Serve over lettuce leaves and season with paprika.

20. Chicken Waldorf Salad

(Ready in about 5 minutes | Serving 4 | Difficulty: Easy)

Per serving: Kcal 224, Fat: 15 g, Net Carbs: 9 g, Protein: 14 g

Ingredients:

- ½ tbsp. ground ginger

- ½ cup chopped apple

- 8 oz. cubed and cooked chicken

- ½ cup Miracle Whip

- ½ cup chopped celery

- 2 tbsp. raisins

Instructions:

1. Blend ingredients together and place in the fridge for some time to let the flavors infuse.

21. Cucumber Cups Stuffed with Buffalo Chicken Salad

(Ready in about 35 minutes | Serving 8 | Difficulty: Easy)

Per serving: Kcal 155, Fat: 13 g, Net Carbs: 3 g, Protein: 18 g

Ingredients:

- 1 tsp. cayenne pepper

- ½ tsp. black pepper

- ½ tsp. Italian seasoning

- 2 tbsp. hot sauce

- ½ cup Kraft® mayonnaise

- 2 large deseeded cucumbers (1" pieces), having half of the center removed

- ¼ cup crumbled blue cheese

- 1 tsp. smoked paprika

- 2 tbsp. lemon juice

- 1 tbsp. chopped fresh garlic

- 2 tbsp. chopped fresh chives

- ¼ cup chopped fresh parsley

- 3 cups shredded chicken breast

Instructions:

1. Except for the cucumbers and chicken, mix everything together. In that mix, add chicken and combine well. Put it in the fridge for around thirty minutes.
2. Then add around 2 tsp. of the mixture to each slice of a cucumber and sprinkle chopped parsley over it.

22. Fall Harvest Orzo Salad

(Ready in about 5 minutes | Serving 8 | Difficulty: Easy)

Per serving: Kcal 289, Fat: 12 g, Net Carbs: 38 g, Protein: 6 g

Ingredients:

- ¼ cup chopped blanched almonds

- 1 cup cranberries dried

- ½ tsp. black pepper

- ¼ cup EVOO

- 4 cups chilled and cooked orzo

- 2 cups diced fresh apples

- ½ cup blue cheese, crumbled

- ¼ cup lemon juice

- 2 tbsp. chopped fresh basil

Instructions:

1. Except for almonds and blue cheese, mix everything together.
2. Transfer it to the serving dish and garnish with almonds and blue cheese.

23. Hawaiian Chicken Salad Sandwich

(Ready in about 5 minutes | Serving 4 | Difficulty: Easy)

Per serving: Kcal 349, Fat: 17 g, Net Carbs: 23 g, Protein: 22 g

Ingredients:

- ½ tsp. black pepper

- 4 flatbread pieces

- ½ cup mayonnaise

- 1 cup tidbits pineapple

- 2 cups cooked chicken

- ½ cup bell pepper

- 1/3 cup carrots

Instructions:

1. Chop the chicken in squares, drain liquid from the pineapple and chop the carrots and bell pepper.
2. Combine all of them and put them in the fridge to chill.
3. Then serve this salad tortilla or bread.

24. Peach, Arugula and Quinoa Salad

(Ready in about 10 minutes | Serving 2 | Difficulty: Easy)

Per serving: Kcal 247, Fat: 7 g, Net Carbs: 32 g, Protein: 8 g

Ingredients:

- 2 fresh medium peaches

- ½ medium bell pepper

- 2 cups arugula

- 1/3 cup quinoa

- 1 fresh shallot

- 2 tbsp. unsalted walnuts

Instructions:

1. Prepare the quinoa as per the directions on the box.

2. Slice the bell pepper and cut the shallot. Halve the peaches and cut the pits. Then have the walnuts sliced.

3. Spray a pan or skillet loosely with oil and heat over moderate flame.

4. Add the walnuts, when finely toasted, to the hot skillet for 1–2 min. Remove and set aside from the pan.

5. In the pan, add peach halves, bell pepper, and shallot. Cook until gently browned and fluffy. Withdraw from the heat.

6. Cover 1 cup arugula with cooked quinoa to assemble the salad. Divide and top each salad with the rest of the ingredients.

7. Serve with your own vinaigrette dressing.

Chapter 6: Fish and Seafood

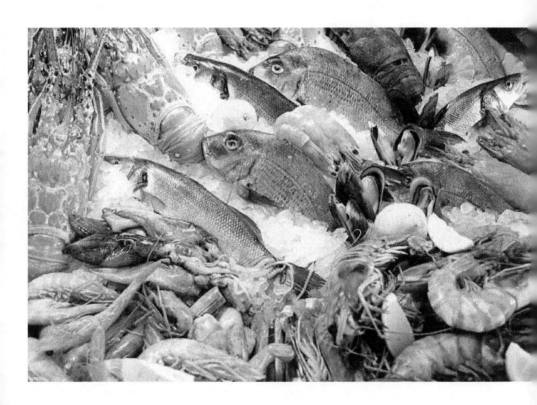

25. Shrimp Scampi

(Ready in about 5 minutes | Serving 4 | Difficulty: Easy)

Per serving: Kcal 265, Fat: 17 g, Net Carbs: 1 g, Protein: 24 g

Ingredients:

- ½ cup white wine

- 5 chopped garlic cloves

- ½ cup butter

- 1 ½ lb. Shrimp

Instructions:

1. Prepare the shrimps and fry the garlic in the butter, then cook till white.
2. After that, add the wine and cook for another five minutes and serve with rice or pasta.

26. Broiled Garlic Shrimp

(Ready in about 15 minutes | Serving 5 | Difficulty: Easy)

Per serving: Kcal 404, Fat: 0 g, Net Carbs: 1 g, Protein: 14 g

Ingredients:

- 2 tbsp. chopped onion

- 1 minced garlic clove

- 2 tsp. lemon juice

- 1 lb. shelled Shrimp

- 1 cup melted unsalted margarine

- 1/8 tsp. pepper

- 1 tbsp. fresh parsley, chopped

Instructions:

1. Preheat the broiler.
2. Clean the shrimp and dry it.
3. Pour the lemon juice, margarine, garlic, onion, and black pepper into a deep baking tray.
4. Attach the shrimp and coat with a flip.
5. For 5 minutes, broil. Five additional minutes, change side and broil.
6. Serve with filtered pan juices on a tray. With parsley, sprinkle.
7. Peel and consume the shrimp.

27. Spring Squid with Pasta and Anchovy Sauce

(Ready in about 15 minutes | Serving 4 | Difficulty: Easy)

Per serving: Kcal 302, Fat: 11 g, Net Carbs: 27 g, Protein: 21 g

Ingredients:

For Sauce:

- 6 filets anchovy
- 2 tbsp. rosemary leaves
- ½ tsp. cumin powder
- 1/3 cup olive oil
- 2 lemons juice

For Pasta with Squid:

- 12 oz. cleaned squid without ink sac
- ½ tbsp. olive oil
- 2 cups cooked orzo
- 1 tbsp. flat-leaf chopped parsley
- 1 cup frozen peas

- 1 dried crumbled red chili

- 1 garlic clove

Instructions:

Sauce:

1. Mince rosemary and place in a mortar and pestle with anchovies and cumin. Grind yourself into a paste.

2. For the use of an electric mixer, put the paste in a food processor or a cylinder.

3. Attach the mixer or cylinder with the rosemary/anchovy combination and lemon juice. Process till blended properly.

4. Apply oil, gently, until it creates a thickened yet pourable sauce.

Pasta with squid:

1. According to box instructions, ready the orzo. Reserve and drain.
2. Score with vertical lines on the flat squid shell, and then render lines the other way again to create a cross-hatch design.
3. Carry the garlic to a boil with a skillet of water. Add peas and cook until tender, for 5 minutes.
4. Stir it into a dish with the slotted spoon. Mix the olive oil with 1 tablespoon.
5. Warm the grill or a plate with a griddle. Using vegetable oil to mist.
6. Cook squid on the hot plate, even the tentacles, side down, then cook about 1–2 mins. Flip over and apply 30 more seconds to cook.
7. Break the squid into parts that are bite-sized Toss together precisely 3 teaspoons of the liquid with the red chili, squid, peas, and anchovy sauce.
8. Over the orzo, serve in plates or small cups. On each part, sprinkle the parsley.

28. Shrimp and Coconut Curry Noodle Bowl

(Ready in about 30 minutes | Serving 5 | Difficulty: Easy)

Per serving: Kcal 418, Fat: 27 g, Net Carbs: 31 g, Protein: 16 g

Ingredients:

- 1 diced sweet onion

- 2 tbsp. coconut oil

- 8 oz. rice noodles

- 2 cobs sweet corn (kernels removed from cob)

- 2 diced summer squash or zucchini

- 2 garlic cloves, minced

- 2 tbsp. Thai curry paste, red

- 1 tbsp. low-sodium soy sauce

- 14 oz. full-fat canned coconut milk

- 1/3 to 1/2 cup water

- ¼ cup chopped fresh cilantro

- 2 tsp. honey

- 1 tbsp. grated fresh ginger

- ½ lime, juiced and zested

- 2 Chopped onions

- 2 Sliced jalapeño

Instructions:

1. Prepare rice noodles as instructed.
2. In a large frying pan, warm coconut oil. Connect the onion and cook for around 5 minutes over high heat. Put the corn, zucchini, ginger, and garlic and simmer for another five minutes or so before it all begins to soften.
3. Mix in the paste with the curry and simmer for the next minute.

4. Add soy sauce, coconut milk, water, and honey to the mixture. Bring the mixture to a boil and simmer until it starts to get dense. When the sauce gets too thick, you should add more water.

5. Withdraw the skillet from the flame. Apply either basil or cilantro and stir in lime zest and juice, depending on the flavor.

6. Split rice noodles in individual bowls for serving and finish with a mixture of curry. **Optional:** Finish with green onions and/or jalapeño peppers, per taste.

Chapter 7: Poultry and Meat

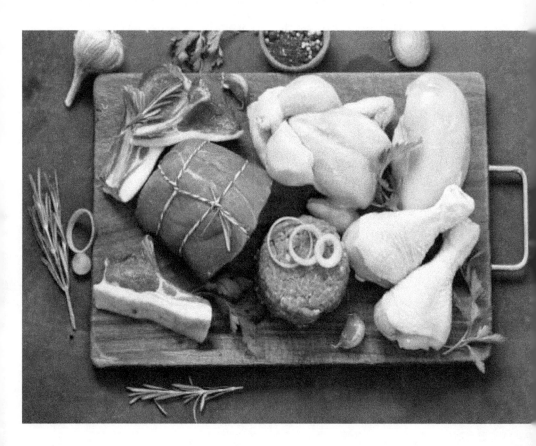

29. Cornish Hens with Tarragon

(Ready in about 80 minutes | Serving 4 | Difficulty: Hard)

Per serving: Kcal 286, Fat: 12 g, Net Carbs: 1 g, Protein: 24 g

Ingredients:

- 1 garlic clove, sliced, pared

- ¼ lb. margarine

- Pepper as per taste

- 1 tbsp. chopped fresh parsley

- 1 tbsp. tarragon

- 2 (1 ¼ lb. each) Cornish hens

Instructions:

1. Cut off the extra skin from the neck and tail fat. Apply garlic on the skin; brush gently with pepper. Put the hens in a 2" shallow baking sheet, skin side up.

2. Warm margarine till it is melted; put tarragon and parsley; fully mix. Bake the hens to 350°F, drizzle them every 15 mins for 1 hour with the tarragon mix. Before eating, drain the margarine.

30. Roasted Red Pepper Pesto

(Ready in about 15 minutes | Serving 2 | Difficulty: Easy)

Per serving: Kcal 526, Fat: 37 g, Net Carbs: 29 g, Protein: 17 g

Ingredients:

- ¼ cup torn fresh basil

- 1 tsp. balsamic vinegar

- 7 oz. roasted drained red peppers

- ¼ cup olive oil

- 2 halved garlic cloves

- 1 tortellini or ravioli

- Pepper as per taste

Instructions:

1. In a blender, mix all ingredients other than the pasta and blend for 30 sec until it has achieved the perfect consistency. Taste and tailor taste to your liking.

2. As per the guidance on the box, cook the stuffed pasta or ravioli. Don't salt pasta water; sauce and ravioli contain a lot of sodium.

3. Cover hot ravioli with room temp pesto instantly and eat it.

31. Rosemary Chicken

(Ready in about 40 minutes | Serving 4 | Difficulty: Medium)

Per serving: Kcal 539, Fat: 32 g, Net Carbs: 20 g, Protein: 37 g

Ingredients:

- 2 tsp. dried and crushed rosemary

- 1/3 cup brown sugar

- ¼ cup sunflower oil

- ¼ cup lime juice

- 1 chicken broiler-fryer (halved)

- ½ cup white wine dry

- 1 tsp. Worcestershire sauce

Instructions:

1. In a shallow dish, combine all the ingredients, excluding chicken, to produce a marinade.
2. Attach the chicken and switch with the marinade to cover. Cover for at minimum 4 hrs and refrigerate, rotating periodically.
3. Drain the chicken, retaining the basting marinade.
4. Place the chicken in a broiling pan around 7–9 inches from the heat source, skin cut side, on the rack. Broil around 20 minutes, basting poultry with marinade on occasion. Turn the chicken, baste and broil generously for 15 minutes or till soft.
5. Dispose of every marinade that stands.

32. Tasty Beef Ribs

(Ready in about 1 hour 30 minutes | Serving 8 | Difficulty: Hard)

Per serving: Kcal 187, Fat: 11 g, Net Carbs: 2 g, Protein: 19 g

Ingredients:

- 1/8 tsp. red pepper

- ¼ cup pineapple juice

- 1 tbsp. paprika

- ¼ tsp. mustard powder

- 4 lb. beef ribs large

- 2 tsp. chili powder

- ½ tsp. garlic powder

Instructions:

1. Put a single line of ribs in 2 deep roasting, meaty cut side on racks pans. Roast for 30 minutes in a 450°F oven. Drain.
2. Rub the pineapple juice through the ribs.
3. Mix the rest of the ingredients together. Sprinkle uniformly on the ribs in both directions.
4. Lower the oven to 350°F. Roast ribs for the next 45–60 min on the meaty side up.

33. Sukiyaki and Rice

(Ready in about 30 minutes | Serving 10 | Difficulty: Easy)

Per serving: Kcal 495, Fat: 29 g, Net Carbs: 31 g, Protein: 24 g

Servings: 10

Ingredients:

- 2 ½ lb. thinly sliced lean beef

- ½ cup celery (½" slices)

- 1 cup white turnip (1/8" slices)

- 1 medium-sized onion (1/8" slices)

- 3 medium thinly sliced scallions

- 2 tbsp. low-sodium soy sauce

- 1 tbsp. water

- 1 medium chopped in rings green pepper

- ¾ cup mushrooms, sliced

- 1 cup cabbage, shredded

- 1 tbsp. vegetable oil

- 1 tbsp. sugar

- 5 cups white rice, cooked

- ½ cup broccoli, chopped, frozen

- 1 sliced tomato, medium

Instructions:

1. Put oil in a wide massive skillet; on both sides, gently brown meat.
2. In order of the recipe list of ingredients, transform heat to boil and bring veggies into the pan (in layers).
3. Combine the sugar, water, and soy sauce; spill over the veggies.
4. Close and steam for 10–15 minutes under low pressure. You don't stir.
5. Present with rice (per meal, half cup rice).

34. Spicy Pork Chops with Apples

(Ready in about 50 minutes | Serving 6 | Difficulty: Medium)

Per serving: Kcal 215, Fat: 13 g, Net Carbs: 10 g, Protein: 15 g

Ingredients:

- 3/4 tsp. salt

- 2 minced, pared garlic cloves

- 1 tsp. ginger powder

- 2 medium-sized cored and unpared apples (1" slices)

- ½ tsp. sugar

- ¼ tsp. cumin powder

- ¼ tsp. pepper

- 1 large pared red onion (¾" slices)

- 6 pork chops large

- Rice (½)cup

Instructions:

1. Mix the six components first.
2. Rub the seasoning mix on every pork chop on both sides.
3. Put it in a wide glass tub.
4. Among chops, insert pieces of apples and onions.
5. Crumple the aluminum foil and press the components together at either end of the plate.
6. Encompass with foil; cook for 20 mins at 400°F.
7. Lower the heat to around 325°F; simmer for 30–35 mins.
8. Reveal. Uncover.
9. To distinguish chops, peel crumpled foil; bake for approximately 15 minutes once light brown.
10. Over rice, eat.

35. Chicken Enchiladas

(Ready in about 80 minutes | Serving 7 | Difficulty: Medium)

Per serving: Kcal 351, Fat: 21 g, Net Carbs: 22 g, Protein: 17 g

Ingredients:

Sauce:

- 2 garlic cloves, minced
- 1 tbsp. olive oil
- 2 tsp. minced parsley
- ½ tsp. dried oregano
- 2 ½ tsp. chili powder
- 1 tsp. minced onion
- 1 cup water
- ½ tsp. black pepper
- ½ tsp. dried basil
- ½ tsp. ground cumin
- 6 oz. no-salt canned tomato sauce

Enchiladas:

- 8 oz. boiled and shredded chicken
- 2 tbsp. canola oil
- 1 medium chopped onion
- 7 oz. diced canned green chilis
- 8 oz. chicken broth low sodium
- 8 oz. sour cream
- 3 chopped green onions
- 7 (6") flour tortillas
- 1 recipe Enchilada sauce
- 1 cup Monterey jack shredded cheese

Instructions:

Sauce:

1. Heat oil over moderate flame in a saucepan. Add the onion and garlic and simmer for two min.
2. Get the rest of the ingredients to a simmer. Continue cooking for 20 minutes, then reduce the flame. Just placed back.

Enchiladas:

1. Preheat your oven to 350°F.
2. Heat oil over moderate heat in a skillet. Garnish with onions and roast for five min.
3. Stir in the chicken, chili peppers, and chicken broth. Boil, raise the heat, and cook for fifteen minutes. Bring to a boil.
4. Combine the sour cream and part of the onions together.
5. Spoon the 1/3 cup mixture of chicken on every tortilla. Roll the tortilla up and put the seam in a 9x9 baking dish in a thin layer. Garnish with the enchilada, cheese, and leftover green onion.
6. For 30 minutes, roast.

36. Honey Garlic Chicken

(Ready in about 65 minutes | Serving 4 | Difficulty: Medium)

Per serving: Kcal 279, Fat: 10 g, Net Carbs: 36 g, Protein: 13 g

Ingredients:

- 1 tbsp. olive oil

- ½ cup honey

- 1 tsp. garlic powder

- ½ tsp. black pepper

- 4 lb. roasting chicken

Instructions:

1. Preheat the oven to 350°F.

2. Oil the baking sheet.

3. Place the chicken in the pan to prevent conflicting bits. Coat the meat with seasonings and butter.

4. Cook for around 1 hr or till all sides are brown. While cooking, switch once.

37. Chili Con Carne and Rice

(Ready in about 1 hour 30 minutes | Serving 7 | Difficulty: Medium)

Per serving: Kcal 260, Fat: 9 g, Net Carbs: 28 g, Protein: 15 g

Ingredients:

- 3 ½ cups cooked rice

- 1 cup onion, chopped

- 1 lb. lean minced beef

- 3 cups water

- 1 cup green pepper, chopped

- 6 oz. no-salt canned tomato paste

- 2 tsp. garlic powder

- 1 tsp. paprika

- 1 tsp. ground cumin

- ½ cup pinto beans cooked (without salt)

Instructions:

1. In a big pan, cook the minced beef and remove excess fat.

2. Combine the onion and green pepper and cook until the onion becomes clear. Add the other ingredients and braise for 1 ½ hrs.

3. Over hot fresh rice, serve.

38. Curried Turkey and Rice

(Ready in about 20 minutes | Serving 6 | Difficulty: Easy)

Per serving: Kcal 154, Fat: 5 g, Net Carbs: 19 g, Protein: 8 g

Ingredients:

- 1 tsp. vegetable oil

- 1 lb. turkey breast (sliced in 8 cutlets)

- 1 medium chopped onion

- 1 tbsp. unsalted margarine

- 2 tsp. curry powder

- 2 tbsp. flour

- 1 cup low-sodium chicken broth

- 2 cups white rice, cooked

- ½ cup non-dairy creamer

- 1 tsp. sugar

Instructions:

1. Heat the oil in a broad skillet. Add turkey. Cook, rotating once before pink, is no longer there around ten minutes. Set the turkey over a plate. To stay warm, wrap in foil.

2. Melt the margarine in the same pan. Apply the chopped onion and curry powder. Cook for five min, stirring. Attach flour when continually stirring.

3. Using broth, creamer, and sugar to blend. Stir regularly until the mixture thickens.

4. Send the turkey back to the skillet. Roast, rotating until warmed, around 2 minutes, to coat.

5. Serve over rice with turkey and sauce.

Chapter 8: Vegetarian

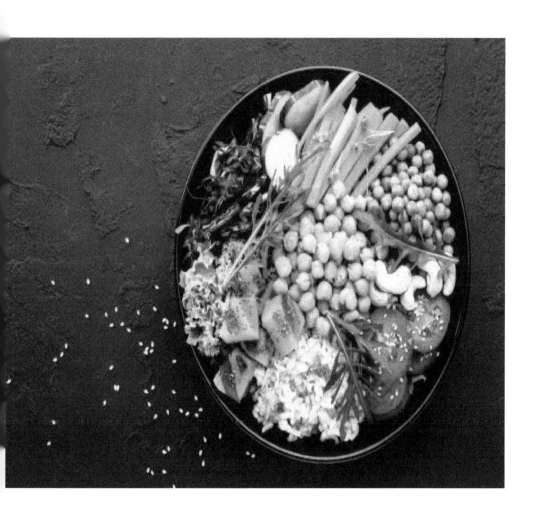

39. Rice Pilaf Baked in a Pumpkin

(Ready in about 1 hour 40 minutes | Serving 8 | Difficulty: Medium)

Per serving: Kcal 460, Fat: 15 g, Net Carbs: 80 g, Protein: 5 g

Ingredients:

- 3 cups without salt cooked rice

- 1 cup fresh or dry cranberries

- 2 tbsp. canola oil

- 2 small diced onions

- 2 peeled and diced carrots

- 2 diced celery stalks

- 2 chopped garlic cloves

- 5 lb. raw pumpkin

Instructions:

1. Pumpkin shell and rice pilaf can be cooked ahead of time and kept separately in the fridge before it's time to place it in the oven.

Preparation of Shells:

1. Cut the top of the pumpkin carefully to prepare the pumpkin casing. When put back on the pumpkin, make sure it would fit snugly. Only set aside.

2. To produce an empty wrapper, clean the interior of the pumpkin. Discard the seeds and the substance inside.

3. Place the entire pumpkin on a cookie sheet or baking tray lined with foil.

Preparation for Filling:

1. You can need to double the rice pilaf ingredients if you have a big pumpkin.

2. If not already created, prepare the rice to create the pilaf filling. In a saucepan, sauté all the veggies in canola oil until they are tender.

3. Stir in the cranberries, seasonings, and rice.

To Bake:

1. Preheat the oven at 350°F.

2. Spoon the rice pilaf softly into the hollow pumpkin shell and replace the pumpkin top to protect it. Put it in a casserole dish if you are not using a pumpkin.

3. Bake for around 60 minutes, or before a fork or knife quickly pierces the pumpkin skin. Cover and bake for just 30 minutes or until completely cooked, if using a casserole dish. 4. Let it cool for 15 minutes at least.

5. Serve warm or at room temperature with a large serving spoon by scooping portions out of pumpkin shell.

6. To make 8 to 12 wedges, slice through the pumpkin for more pleasure. Serve alongside the pilaf with a wedge. It'll make the pumpkin tender but strong. Eat just the pumpkin flesh and detach the thick skin.

40. Black Bean Burger and Cilantro Slaw

(Ready in about 15 minutes | Serving 6 | Difficulty: Easy)

Per serving: Kcal 380, Fat: 19 g, Net Carbs: 40 g, Protein: 9 g

Ingredients:

- 1 tsp. black pepper

- ½ cup drained, rinsed, dried and mashed black beans

- 1 tsp. granulated garlic

- ½ tsp. smoked paprika

- 1 tsp. onion flakes

- ½ cup of bulgur wheat

- 1 tbsp. reduced-sodium Worcestershire sauce

- ¼ cup of scallions

- 1 tbsp. reduced-sodium beef base

- 2 tbsp. flour

- ½ cup sautéed onions, until translucent

- 1 zested lime

- 3 cups slaw mix

- 2 tbsp. canola oil

- 2 tbsp. sesame oil

- 6 rolls hamburger

- ¼ cup balsamic vinegar

- ¼ cup mayonnaise

- 2 tbsp. cilantro

- ¼ cup lime juice

Instructions:

1. Preheat the oven at 400°F.
2. Combine bulgur wheat, granular garlic, black pepper, beef bouillon, Worcestershire sauce, black beans, onion

flakes, smoked paprika, onion, and half a cup of scallions in a standard size dish.

3. Mold about half a cup of the mix into burgers and freeze (but not frozen).

4. Create a vinaigrette by combining 1 tbsp. of cilantro, lime juice, sesame oil and vinegar together. Apply all but 2 tbsp. of vinaigrette to the slaw mix in a small bowl and whisk gently, then put aside in the refrigerator.

5. Add the mayo and the leftover 2 tbsp. of vinaigrette to another tiny bowl and put aside.

6. Dust the flour on the black bean burgers and scrape the waste. Put on the pre-sprayed pan and also spray the burger tops. Cook about 14 minutes, then flip around midway through the burgers.

7. Toast rolls and distributes equivalent volumes of mayo. Attach the black bean burger and cover with around ¼ of a cup (or the quantity you want of slaw).

41. Grilled Multicolored Peppers and Onions

(Ready in about 20 minutes | Serving 4 | Difficulty: Easy)

Per serving: Kcal 154, Fat: 13 g, Net Carbs: 9 g, Protein: 1 g

Ingredients:

- 1 Vidalia onion, medium

- ¼ tsp. salt

- ¾ tsp. black pepper

- 1 each red, yellow and green bell pepper

- 1/3 cup olive oil

- 1 red onion, medium

Instructions:

1. Quarter-cut all onions together. Peppers are seeded and sliced into 8 parts.
2. For specific grilling, plan the protected grill.
3. Combine all the ingredients in a wide tub, tossing properly enough that the veggies are covered equally with oil.
4. Put the veggies in a basket for a grill. Grill for around 18 minutes, sometimes turning the veggies on all sides to brown uniformly.

42. Crunchy Green Bean Casserole

(Ready in about 25 minutes | Serving 6 | Difficulty: Easy)

Per serving: Kcal 122, Fat: 6 g, Net Carbs: 8 g, Protein: 4 g

Ingredients:

- 12 oz. green beans

- ½ cup crushed unsalted, plain tortilla chips

- ¼ cup crumbled gorgonzola

- 2 tbsp. melted, unsalted butter

- 2 tbsp. hot sauce

- ½ cup breadcrumbs

- 2 tbsp. chopped green onions

Instructions:

1. Preheat the oven at 375°F.
2. Cut green beans into ~2" bits (steam in an oven plate for 5–7 mins, wet damp paper towel).
3. Combine the hot sauce with the sliced string of green beans. Dump the combination into the casserole bowl.
4. In a small cup, blend the remaining ingredients. Scatter mixture uniformly across string beans, then bake uncovered bean casserole in the oven for 15 minutes or till crispness is desired, then serve.

Chapter 9: Desserts

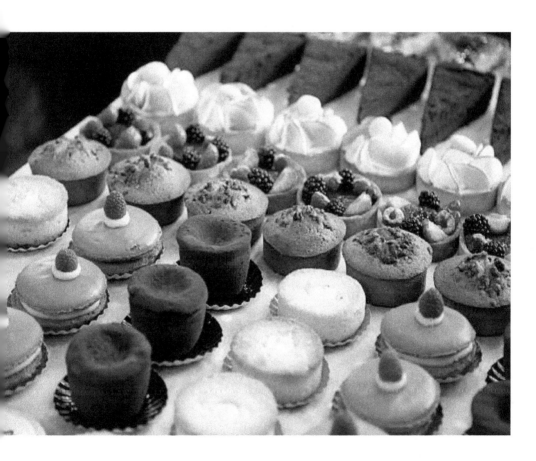

43. Pineapple Salsa

(Ready in about 10 minutes | Serving 16 | Difficulty: Easy)

Per serving: Kcal 16, Fat: 0 g, Net Carbs: 4 g, Protein: 0 g

Ingredients:

- 2 tbsp. cilantro

- ¼ cup onion

- 1 garlic clove

- 10 oz. juice-packed pineapple tidbits, canned

- 1 tbsp. jalapeño pepper

Instructions:

1. The garlic, onion and jalapeno are minced. Cilantro chop.
2. Place the pineapple in a non-reactive pot and rinse.
3. Other components are applied and combine properly.

4. For mixing flavors, refrigerate for many hours in the fridge.

44. Pumpkin Strudel

(Ready in about 30 minutes | Serving 8 | Difficulty: Easy)

Per serving: Kcal 180, Fat: 8 g, Net Carbs: 23 g, Protein: 3 g

Ingredients:

- 1 tsp. extract pure vanilla

- 1½ cup sodium-free, canned pumpkin, unsweetened

- 12 phyllo dough sheets

- 4 tbsp. sugar

- 1/8 tsp. grated nutmeg

- ½ tsp. cinnamon powder

- 4 tbsp. melted, unsalted butter

Instructions:

1. In the center of the oven, place the oven rack. Preheat the furnace to 375°F.

2. Mix the packaged pumpkin, vanilla extract, nutmeg, 2 tbsp. of sugar and 1/2 tbsp. of cinnamon in a medium-sized bowl until well combined.

3. Cover the base of the nonstick moderate tray with the molten butter using a pastry tool. Put a single layer of phyllo dough on a smooth work surface and grease with butter. Brush phyllo sheet using butter, then build a pile of phyllo sheets. Hold the leftover plastic wrap-covered phyllo sheets ready to be used, so they do not dry out.

4. Spoon the mixture uniformly over one of the stack's long edges until all sheets are utilized. Roll to the unfilled side from the loaded end so that the crease faced down.

5. Switch the roll to the seam-side-down oiled sheet tray and spray with the leftover butter.

6. Blend the leftover sugar and cinnamon in a shallow dish. Toss over the strudel's top and bottom.

7. Bake until toasted or lightly browned on the middle rack, around 15 mins.

8. Prior to slicing using a sharp knife, remove the tray from the oven and let the crispy strudel to sit for 10 minutes, enabling the core to settle. Then serve.

45. Rustic Apple Cinnamon Filled Phyllo Pastries

(Ready in about 35 minutes | Serving 6 | Difficulty: Easy)

Per serving: Kcal 280, Fat: 13 g, Net Carbs: 33 g, Protein: 2 g

Ingredients:

Apple mixture:

- ¼ cup sugar light brown

- 1 tsp. cinnamon

- 2 tbsp. firm butter, unsalted

- ¼ tsp. cornstarch

- ¼ cup melted butter, unsalted

- ¼ tsp. nutmeg

- 6 phyllo dough sheets

- 2 tbsp. vanilla extract

- 4 diced apples

In a small bowl, mix:

- 2 tbsp. cinnamon

- 3 tbsp. powdered sugar

For garnish:

- Powdered sugar

- Whipped cream

- Mint sprigs

Instructions:

Apple mixture:

1. Preheat the oven at 350°F.

2. Sauté the apples in the butter for 6–8 minutes in a wide saucepan over medium heat.

3. Stir in the cinnamon, brown sugar, and nutmeg. Cook for 3 or 4 more minutes.

4. Mix the cornstarch and vanilla essence in a tiny cup before it is depleted. Stir in the apple blend and simmer on a moderate flame for an extra two mins.

5. Switch off the heat and set aside the mixture.

Phyllo Pastries:

1. A big 6-muffin pan tin is loosely greased.

2. Wipe each surface with butter and then sprinkle with the icing sugar and cinnamon combination, beginning with the first layer of phyllo dough. Continue till all 6 sheets of sugar and cinnamon blend have buttered and dusted, piling layer by layer.

3. Break the stack into 6 pieces each. Using one set of squares to line the base and sides

of every muffin cup, leaving several of the squares dangling over the sides of muffin cups.

4. Load the apple blend in every phyllo-lined cup of muffin midway to 3 qt. complete (this depends on how wide the apples were sliced), meaning that every phyllo-lined cup of the muffin has equivalent quantities of apple blend.
5. In muffin cups, fold the extra phyllo dough at apples.
6. Bake till light golden in the preheated oven around 350°F.

46. Very Berry Bread Pudding

(Ready in about 60 minutes | Serving 10 | Difficulty: Medium)

Per serving: Kcal 392, Fat: 23 g, Net Carbs: 34 g, Protein: 9 g

Ingredients:

- 1 tbsp. orange zest

- 6 beaten eggs

- 8 cups challah bread, cubed

- 2 cups heavy cream

- 12 oz. thawed berry medley

- ½ cup sugar

- Whipped cream (½ cup)

- 2 tsp. vanilla

- ½ tsp. cinnamon

Instructions:

1. Preheat oven at 375°F.
2. Whisk together the orange zest, eggs, cream, sugar, cinnamon and vanilla till tender.
3. Mix the cubes of bread and the fruit with your hands.
4. Put into a buttered tray and bake for about thirty minutes, filled with tape. Ensure that it is unsalted before using butter.
5. Take the foil and cook for an extra 15 minutes.
6. Switch the oven off and let the oven stay for ten min.
7. Slice, then eat with cream on top.

47. Sunburst Lemon Bars

(Ready in about 45 minutes | Serving 24 | Difficulty: Medium)

Per serving: Kcal 200, Fat: 9 g, Net Carbs: 28 g, Protein: 2 g

Ingredients:

Crust:

- 1 cup unsalted butter at room temperature

- ½ cup sugar, powdered

- 2 cups white flour

Filling:

- ¼ cup lemon juice

- 4 eggs

- ¼ tsp. baking soda

- 1½ cup sugar

- ¼ cup white flour

- ½ tsp. tartar cream

Glaze:

- 2 tbsp. lemon juice

- 1 cup sifted powdered sugar

Instructions:

Crust:

1. Preheat the oven at 350°F.
2. Mix the flour, icing sugar and softened butter in a wide dish. Mix together until crumbly. In a 9" by 13" baking sheet, push the mixture onto the rim.
3. Bake for around 15 to 20 minutes, until nicely browned.

Filling:

1. Whisk the eggs gently in a moderate dish.
2. Combine the rice, starch, tartar cream, and baking soda in another dish. For the chickens, apply the dry mixture. To the mixture of egg, apply lemon juice and stir until gently thickened.
3. Place over the heated crust and simmer for an additional 20 mins or till set.
4. Remove and cool after taking out from the oven.

Glaze:

1. Mix lemon juice steadily into the sieve powdered sugar in a small bowl until it is spreadable. As desired, add lemon juice.
2. Distribute over the filling that has been cooled. Then let glaze settle and split into 24 bars afterward. Preserve the spare lemon bars in the freezer.

48. Chewy Lemon-Ginger-Coconut Cookies

(Ready in about 25 minutes | Serving 24 | Difficulty: Easy)

Per serving: Kcal 97, Fat: 6 g, Net Carbs: 11 g, Protein: 1 g

Ingredients:

- ½ cup sugar

- 1 egg

- 1 cup unsweetened toasted coconut

- 2 tbsp. lemon juice

- 1 tbsp. lemon zest

- ½ tsp. baking soda

- 1 tbsp. chopped fresh ginger

- 1¼ cup flour

- ½ cup butter unsalted

Instructions:

1. Preheat the oven at 350°F.

2. Scattered sugar-free coconut on the baking tray sheet and bake for around 5-10 minutes until the edges are brown.

3. Take it out of the oven and put it aside in a dish.

4. Cream both sugar and butter until smooth and creamy using an electric mixer. Apply the lemon juice, egg, lemon zest and minced ginger and blend until fluffy.

5. Sift the flour and the baking soda together. In the butter blend, add the flour mix and combine until fully mixed.

6. For a minimum of 30 minutes, cover and relax.

7. Scoop out balls that are tbsp.-size and wrap them within the toasted coconut. Using a loosely oiled baking tray sheet to put balls at minimum 2" apart.

8. Bake for 12 minutes till the sides are softly orange. Detach and cool on the counter.

49. Dried Cranberry Fruit Bars

(Ready in about 50 minutes | Serving 24 | Difficulty: Medium)

Per serving: Kcal 190, Fat: 7 g, Net Carbs: 30 g, Protein: 2 g

Ingredients:

Crust:

- ¾ cup butter, unsalted

- 1 1/3 cup sugar

- 1 ½ cups white flour

Topping:

- ¾ cup sugar

- ½ cup white flour

- 1 tsp. baking powder

- 4 eggs

- 1 cup cranberries, dried

- For dusting powdered sugar (optional)

- 1 tsp. vanilla extract

Instructions:

1. Preheat the oven at 350°F.
2. Stir together the flour and sugar in a small bowl; slice in butter till the mixture sticks together. Tap into the 9" by 13" ungreased baking tray. Bake until gently browned, for 10 minutes.
3. In a shallow cup, sift the baking powder and flour together to create the topping. Throw the dried cranberries in. Just set aside.
4. Mix the eggs, sugar and vanilla in a standard size dish. Apply a blend of flour. Pour the cooked crust onto it. For 20–25 mins, bake.
5. While wet, cut into 24 pieces and sprinkle with icing sugar.

50. Molten Mint Chocolate Brownies

(Ready in about 45 minutes | Serving 12 | Difficulty: Medium)

Per serving: Kcal 307, Fat: 18 g, Net Carbs: 36 g, Protein: 3 g

Ingredients:

- 12 mint chocolates by Andes®

- 1 box brownie mix Betty Crocker® (not supreme)

For garnish:

- Mint sprigs

- Powdered sugar

- Cocoa powder

Instructions:

1. Preheat the oven and prep brownie mix as per the box's guidance.
2. Prepare a lining or finely greased 12 muffin pan and dust the sides and bottom. Through the bowls, put brownie mix and cook for 25 mins.
3. Place one slice of mint candy at the center and cook for an extra five min. Remove the brownies from the oven. Switch the oven off and take it. For 10 min, let cool.
4. Take the brownie cupcakes out of the tray, then serve.

Conclusion

It is known that good eating habits are related to a healthy body. For keeping your kidneys in optimal conditions, you need to choose the proper ingredients that provide the nutrients that help to reduce the risk of renal diseases.

The Kidney-Friendly Diet is the one you need to develop a healthy lifestyle and also enjoy Delicious recipes.

9 781801 563277